MANAGING CHRONIC PAIN NATURALLY:

Holistic Approaches and Alternative therapies that help you get back to the life you love

LEONARD J. GREEN

DISCLAIMER

<u>FREE BONUS GIFT INSIDE THIS BOOK</u>

As a show of appreciation to my readers for purchasing this book I am giving:

A WELL PREPARE DIET PLAN FOR PAIN RELIEVING

TABLE OF CONTENT

Contents

DISCLAIMER 2

INTRODUCTION 7

Acquiring Knowledge of Chronic Pain 7

An explanation of chronic pain 8

Chronic Pain's Impact on Daily Life 9

Why Holistic Approaches and Alternative Therapies Matter 10

CHAPTER 1 12

THE MIND-BODY CONNECTION 12

Exploring the Relationship Between Mind and Body in Pain Management ...12

Mindfulness, Meditation, and Relaxation Techniques 14

Cognitive-behavioral therapy for chronic pain.....................15

CHAPTER 2 17

NUTRITION AND DIET FOR PAIN RELIEF...............17

The Role of Inflammation in Chronic Pain 17

Anti-inflammatory foods and supplements 18

Creating a Pain-Relieving Diet Plan 21

A WELL PREPARE DIET PLAN FOR PAIN RELIEVING.......................23

CHAPTER 3..28

EXERCISE AND MOVEMENT THERAPIES 28

Gentle exercise for chronic pain relief 29

Yoga and Tai Chi for flexibility and strength.................................30

Physical Therapy Techniques for Pain Management 31

CHAPTER 4...33

HERBAL REMEDIES AND NATURAL SUPPLEMENTS 33

An overview of herbal medicine for pain relief 34

Commonly Used Herbs and Their Benefits...................................34

Safety considerations and proper use of herbal remedies.............39

CHAPTER 5...40

ACUPUNCTURE AND ACUPRESSURE 40

Understanding Traditional Chinese Medicine (TCM) Principles...................41

Acupuncture: How It Works and What to Expect.........................42

Acupressure Techniques for Pain Relief at Home.........................43

CHAPTER 6...45

MASSAGE THERAPY AND BODYWORK...........................45

Benefits of Massage for Chronic Pain Management 46

Different types of massage techniques 47

Incorporating Self-Massage into Your Pain Management Routine.................48

CHAPTER 7...50

CHIROPRACTIC ACRE AND SPINAL MANIPULATION 50

The Role of Chiropractic Care in Pain Management......................51

Spinal Manipulation Techniques and Their Efficacy 52

Finding a Qualified Chiropractor and Understanding Treatment Options 53

CHAPTER 8...55

HEAT AND COLD THERAPY 55

Using Heat and Cold to Alleviate Pain and Inflammation 56

Techniques for safe and effective heat and cold therapy.................57

Integrating Heat and Cold into Your Pain Management Plan 58

CHAPTER 9...60

AROMATHERAPY AND ESSENTIALS OILS 60

Introduction to Aromatherapy and Its Benefits 61

Popular essential oils for pain relief...62

Incorporating aromatherapy into your daily routine.......................64

CHAPTER 10 67

MIND-BODY PRACTICES FOR PAIN RELIEF 67

Biofeedback and neurofeedback techniques.....................................68

Guided Imagery and Visualization Exercises..................................69

Hypnotherapy for Pain Management 70

CONCLUSION 72

INTRODUCTION

Acquiring Knowledge of Chronic Pain

Chronic pain is not only a physical sensation; rather, it is an all-encompassing experience that affects all parts of a person's life. It is the unrelenting pain that does not go away the continuous companion that follows every action and thought that makes it difficult to function normally. In this introduction, we will begin our adventure to unravel the complexities of chronic pain.

We will delve into its description, its deep impact on daily existence, and the compelling reasons why it is essential to embrace holistic approaches and alternative therapies in order to regain a life that is full of joy and vitality.

An explanation of chronic pain

When compared to acute pain, chronic pain is not a brief experience that is brought on by an accident or illness; rather, it is a condition that lasts for a long period of time, which can last for weeks, months, or even years. It extends beyond the confines of time, becoming a constant presence in the lives of individuals who struggle to overcome its unrelenting hold on them.

Every form of chronic pain is just as incapacitating as the next, ranging from slow, persistent aches to intense, stabbing sensations. Chronic pain can present in a variety of ways. But the physical agony is not the only thing that defines chronic pain; the emotional toll, the mental misery, and the profound disturbance it inflicts upon one's well-being are the things that truly characterize the essence of chronic pain.

<u>Chronic Pain's Impact on Daily Life</u>

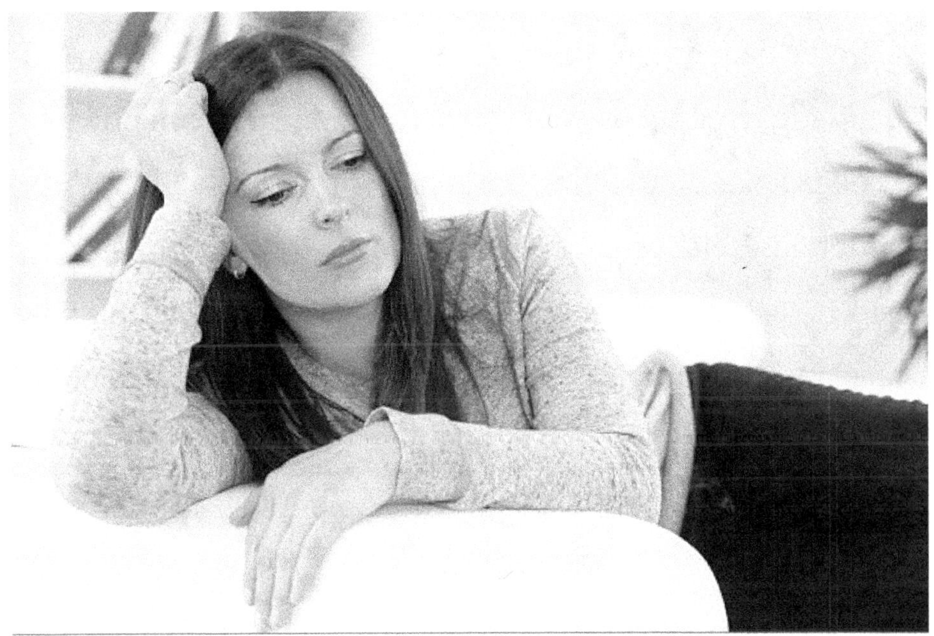

Just try to picture yourself waking up every morning to the same old sensation of misery, knowing that another day of battling unrelenting pain is waiting for you. Simple acts once taken for granted walking, sitting, even sleeping become onerous endeavors, overshadowed by the pervasive anguish that gnaws at the very center of one's existence.

Chronic pain doesn't discriminate; it infiltrates every part of daily life, eroding physical power, diminishing emotional resilience, and shrouding the smallest joys in a veil of suffering. Relationships strain under its weight; jobs suffer; and goals shrink in its shadow. The impact is powerful, far-reaching, and frequently alienating, leaving those afflicted feeling stuck in a prison of their own bodies.

<u>Why Holistic Approaches and Alternative Therapies Matter</u>

Amidst the sorrow and frustration of chronic pain, there lurks a glimmer of hope a path less traveled yet filled with potential. Holistic approaches and alternative therapies offer an alternative narrative that exceeds the limitations of mainstream medicine to address the fundamental causes of suffering and promote healing from within.

Unlike pharmaceutical interventions that only mask symptoms, holistic modalities embrace the interconnectedness of mind, body, and spirit, creating a complete approach to wellness that empowers individuals to recover agency over their health.

CHAPTER 1

THE MIND-BODY CONNECTION

In the field of chronic pain management, the subtle interplay between mind and body emerges as a critical focal point. This chapter goes on a journey to explore the fundamental relationship between mental and physical well-being, investigating the transforming impact of mindfulness meditation, relaxation techniques, and cognitive-behavioral therapy in easing the burden of chronic pain.

<u>Exploring the Relationship Between Mind and Body in Pain Management</u>

At the heart of chronic pain lies a complex web of physiological, psychological, and emotional elements, each impacting the other in a delicate dance of interconnection.

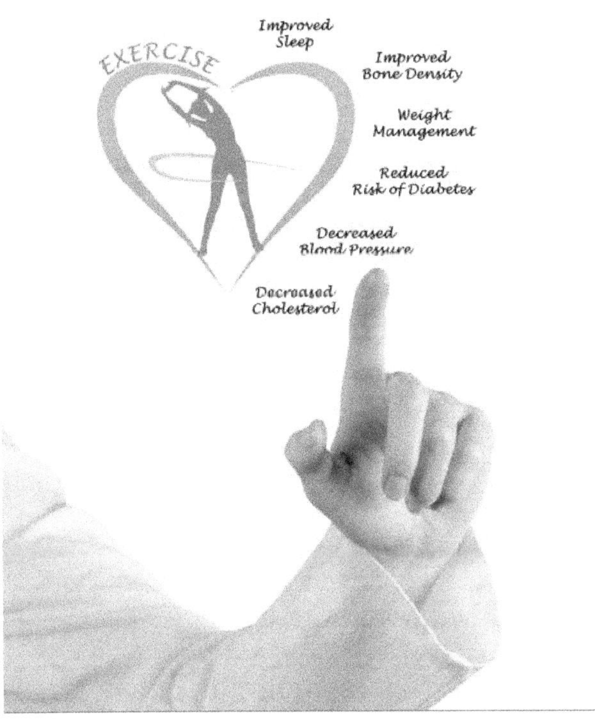

The mind-body connection, formerly rejected as mere supposition, today sits at the forefront of pain management paradigms, offering a comprehensive approach that surpasses the boundaries of traditional interventions. Research underlines the tremendous impact of psychological states on pain perception, with stress, worry, and depression worsening symptoms and prolonging the cycle of suffering. By appreciating the fundamental relationship between mind and body, individuals gain insight into the mechanisms underlying their pain, paving the way for tailored interventions that address the root causes of their suffering.

Mindfulness, Meditation, and Relaxation Techniques

In the tempest of chronic pain, seeking peace amidst the storm may seem like an overwhelming endeavor. Yet, mindfulness meditation and relaxation practices emerge as beacons of hope, offering shelter in the midst of chaos. Rooted in ancient contemplative practices, mindfulness urges individuals to build present-moment awareness, fostering a sense of acceptance and equanimity in the face of adversity. Practitioners learn to attune to the subtle subtleties of feeling, releasing resistance and embracing the body's inherent wisdom through gentle breathwork, body scans, and guided imagery. Likewise, relaxation techniques such as progressive muscle relaxation, autogenic training, and guided imagery give respite from the persistent grip of pain, enabling patients to tap into the body's intrinsic capacity for healing and restoration.

Cognitive-behavioral therapy for chronic pain

As the cliché goes, "Change your thoughts, and you change your world." Nowhere is this attitude more powerful than in the domain of cognitive-behavioral treatment (CBT) for chronic pain. Grounded in the principles of cognitive restructuring and behavioral modification, CBT helps individuals to challenge maladaptive thought patterns, create coping strategies, and reclaim agency over their pain experience. Through controlled sessions with skilled therapists, individuals learn to identify and fight problematic thinking distortions, replacing them with adaptive beliefs that encourage resilience and empowerment. Behavioral approaches such as activity pacing, goal setting, and relaxation training complement cognitive therapies, offering practical solutions for reducing pain-related discomfort and boosting quality of life.

In the pages that follow, we go deeper into the transformative potential of mindfulness meditation, relaxation techniques, and cognitive-behavioral therapy, investigating their use in the context of chronic pain management. Through personal experiences, scientific insights, and practical exercises, readers are inspired to embark on a journey of self-discovery, resilience, and healing, harnessing the power of the mind-body connection to transcend the restrictions of pain and recover a life of vitality and well-being.

CHAPTER 2

NUTRITION AND DIET FOR PAIN RELIEF

Amidst the maze of chronic pain, nutrition emerges as a light of hope, offering a path towards relief and repair. In this chapter, we explore the delicate relationship between diet and pain, delving into the mechanics of inflammation, investigating the therapeutic potential of anti-inflammatory foods and supplements, and building tailored meal regimens aimed to reduce discomfort and increase well-being.

The Role of Inflammation in Chronic Pain

At the heart of many chronic pain disorders lies the sinister specter of inflammation, a complicated immunological reaction that may wreak havoc on the body's delicate equilibrium. Inflammation, marked by redness, swelling, heat, and discomfort, acts as the body's primary defense against damage and infection. However, when inflammation becomes chronic and dysregulated, it can contribute to a plethora of health conditions, including arthritis, fibromyalgia, and autoimmune illnesses. Understanding the function of inflammation in chronic pain is crucial to establishing successful dietary solutions for pain treatment. By targeting underlying inflammatory processes through tailored nutrition interventions, individuals can decrease pain symptoms and boost their overall quality of life.

Anti-inflammatory foods and supplements

In the quest for pain relief, nature offers a cornucopia of anti-inflammatory companions, each filled with the potential to temper the flames of inflammation and restore equilibrium to the body. From vivid fruits and vegetables overflowing with

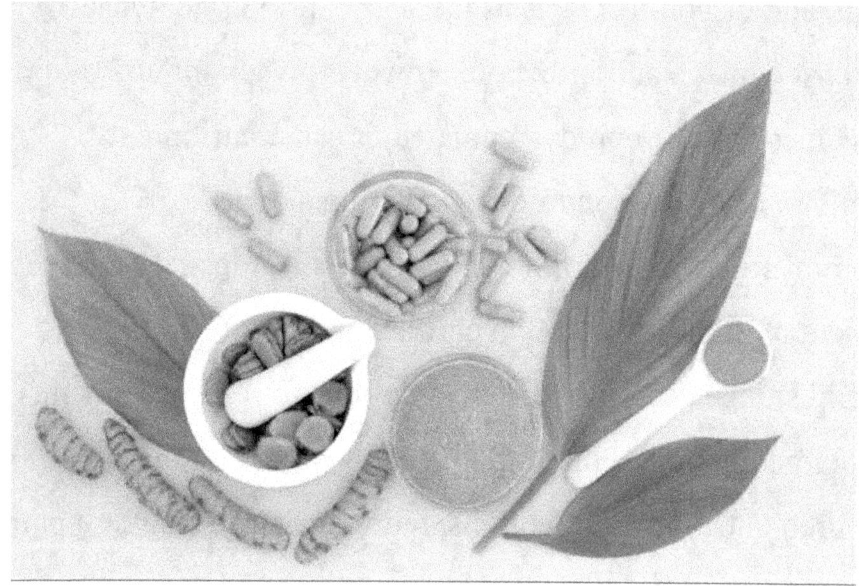

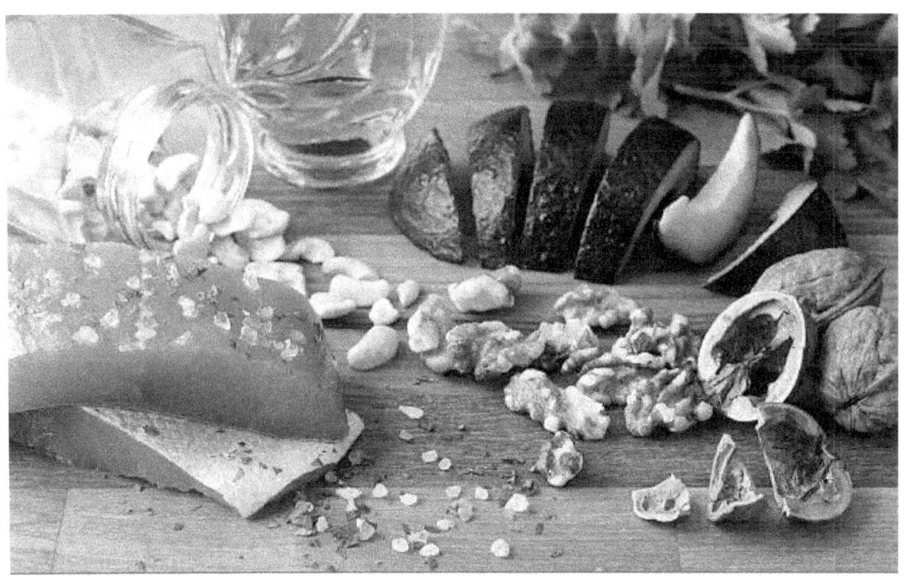

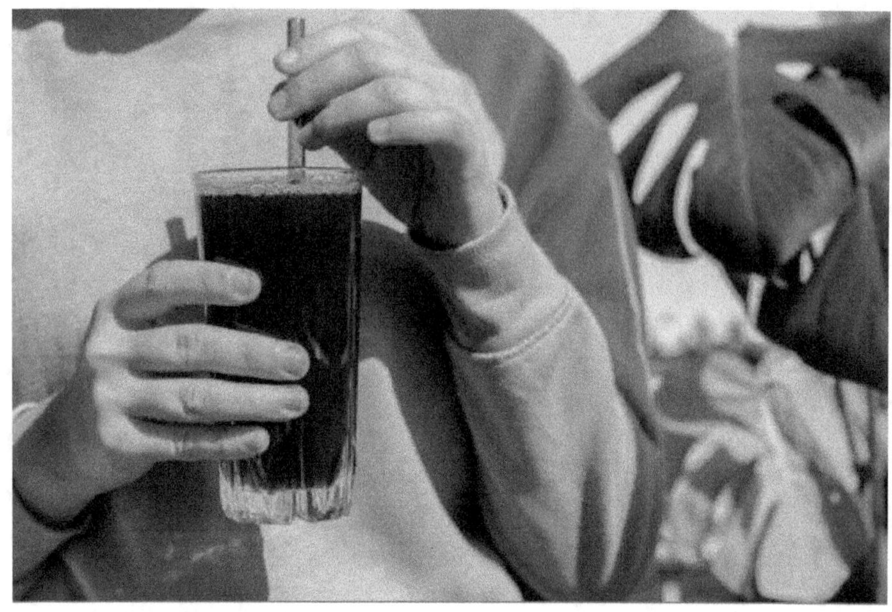

phytonutrients to omega-3 fatty acid-rich fish and nuts, the palette of anti-inflammatory meals is as wide as it is delightful. Turmeric, recognized for its significant anti-inflammatory qualities, includes curcumin, a bioactive molecule that suppresses inflammatory pathways and alleviates pain. Likewise, ginger, green tea, and dark leafy greens offer significant defenses against chronic inflammation, enhancing the body's resilience and vigor.

Supplements, too, play a crucial role in the anti-inflammatory arsenal, delivering tailored support for pain reduction and recovery. Omega-3 fatty acids, contained in fish oil supplements, demonstrate powerful anti-inflammatory actions, regulating immune responses and lowering pain intensity in chronic illnesses such as rheumatoid arthritis and osteoarthritis. Similarly, vitamin D supplementation has been demonstrated to relieve musculoskeletal discomfort and promote general well-being, particularly in those with vitamin D insufficiency. By integrating specific supplements into their daily regimen, individuals can boost the anti-inflammatory advantages of their food and optimize their pain management outcomes.

Creating a Pain-Relieving Diet Plan

Armed with the knowledge of inflammation's involvement in chronic pain and the therapeutic potential of anti-inflammatory foods and supplements, individuals can embark on a path of dietary transformation, constructing tailored meal plans aimed to nourish the body, soothe the soul, and ease pain.

Drawing inspiration from Mediterranean and plant-based diets, which emphasize full, unprocessed foods rich in fruits, vegetables, legumes, and lean proteins, individuals can establish dietary patterns that promote healing and resilience. By prioritizing nutrient-dense foods, minimizing inflammatory triggers such as refined sugars and processed fats, and incorporating targeted supplements as needed, individuals can harness the power of nutrition to reclaim control over their pain experience and embark on a path towards greater vitality and well-being.

A WELL PREPARE DIET PLAN FOR PAIN RELIEVING

Good morning:

Greens such as spinach, kale, pineapple, ginger, turmeric, and coconut water should be blended together to make an anti-inflammatory smoothie. To increase the amount of protein and creaminess in the dish, add a scoop of protein powder or Greek yogurt.

Midmorning Lunch or Snack:

Mixed Berries with Almonds: Take a handful of mixed berries, which may include blueberries, strawberries, and raspberries, and combine them with a handful of almonds. Berries include a high concentration of antioxidants, whereas almonds are a good source of protein and healthy fats.

It's lunchtime:

To make a salad with salmon, combine grilled salmon with mixed greens, avocado, cherry tomatoes, and cucumber. Drizzle the salad with olive oil and balsamic vinegar just before serving. Salmon is an excellent source of omega-3 fatty acids, which are well-known for their ability to reduce inflammation.

Snack in the afternoon:

Greek Yogurt with Honey and Walnuts: Choose plain Greek yogurt with a drizzle of honey and a sprinkling of walnuts. Greek yogurt is abundant in protein, while walnuts contain omega-3 fatty acids.

Dinner:

Quinoa Stir-Fry with Vegetables and Tofu/Chicken: Cook quinoa and stir-fry it with a mix of colorful veggies, such as bell peppers, broccoli, carrots, and snap peas. Add tofu or grilled chicken for protein. Flavor with garlic, ginger, and a dab of low-sodium soy sauce or tamari.

Evening Snack (Optional):

Chamomile Tea with Whole Grain Crackers and Hummus: Enjoy a cup of relaxing chamomile tea alongside whole grain crackers and hummus. Chamomile tea can help encourage relaxation, while whole-grain crackers provide fiber and hummus offers protein.

Hydration:

Drink plenty of water throughout the day. Herbal teas, such as ginger or turmeric tea, can also be calming and hydrating.

General Guidelines:

Emphasize entire, minimally processed foods such as fruits, vegetables, whole grains, lean meats, and healthy fats.

Limit Inflammatory Foods: Reduce intake of processed foods, refined carbohydrates, saturated and trans fats, and excessive alcohol, as they might contribute to inflammation.

Include sources of omega-3 fatty acids, such as fatty fish (salmon, mackerel, and sardines), flaxseeds, chia seeds,

and walnuts.

Use Anti-Inflammatory Spices: Incorporate herbs and spices like turmeric, ginger, garlic, and cinnamon, known for their anti-inflammatory effects.

Practice mindful eating by paying attention to hunger and fullness signs and relishing each bite.

Remember, everyone's body responds differently to foods, so it's vital to listen to your body and adapt the meal plan based on your specific needs and tastes.

Consulting with a healthcare physician or a qualified dietitian can also provide specific guidance for controlling pain through food.

CHAPTER 3

EXERCISE AND MOVEMENT THERAPIES

In the fabric of chronic pain care, the thread of exercise and movement weaves a narrative of perseverance, empowerment, and transformation. In this chapter, we begin on a trip into the domain of gentle exercise, investigating the therapeutic effects of yoga, Tai Chi, and physical therapy techniques in reducing pain, boosting mobility, and cultivating holistic well-being.

From the tranquil embrace of yoga's attentive movements to the graceful cadence of Tai Chi's ancient forms and the targeted interventions of physical therapy, we uncover routes to emancipation from the limitations of pain, inviting movement to become a sanctuary of healing and repair.

Gentle exercise for chronic pain relief

In the loving embrace of gentle exercise, individuals find refuge from the tempest of chronic pain, as movement becomes a catalyst for healing and transformation. Gentle exercises, defined by low-impact motions and attentive awareness, offer a safe and accessible outlet for people seeking relief from pain while cultivating the body's intrinsic ability for recovery.

Walking, swimming, and cycling appear as gentle giants in the field of chronic pain therapy, giving cardiovascular benefits, boosting mood, and promoting overall well-being without exacerbating pain symptoms. By embracing the concept of "start low, go slow," individuals can embark on a path of moderate exercise, acknowledging their body's particular requirements and limits while gradually increasing strength, flexibility, and endurance.

Yoga and Tai Chi for flexibility and strength.

In the exquisite dances of yoga and Tai Chi, individuals discover a sanctuary of silence and movement, where breath and body merge in a symphony of healing and rebirth. Rooted in ancient wisdom and mindfulness practices, yoga and Tai Chi offer substantial advantages for people living with chronic pain, strengthening flexibility, strength, and inner resilience while generating a sense of peace and tranquility.

Through gentle stretches, flowing sequences, and attentive breathwork, individuals can release tension, improve posture, and lessen pain symptoms, establishing a deeper connection with their body and spirit. Whether flowing through a sun salutation in the warmth of a yoga class or gliding through the slow, purposeful movements of Tai Chi in a serene park, individuals find consolation in the embrace of these ancient disciplines, discovering emancipation from the restrictions of pain and limitation.

Physical Therapy Techniques for Pain Management

In the professional hands of physical therapists, clients find partners in their path towards pain alleviation, rehabilitation, and restoration. Physical therapy approaches, ranging from manual therapy and joint mobilization to therapeutic exercises and modalities, offer focused therapies meant to address the underlying causes of pain, enhance mobility, and promote functional independence.

Through specific treatment programs suited to each individual's unique requirements and goals, physical therapists empower clients to retake control over their pain experience, guiding them through a full continuum of care that extends from pain management to long-term wellbeing. By developing a collaborative collaboration between therapist and patient, physical therapy becomes a light of hope and healing, blazing the route towards a life of vitality, resilience, and joy.

CHAPTER 4

HERBAL REMEDIES AND NATURAL SUPPLEMENTS

In the green garden of nature's pharmacy lies a treasure trove of herbal treatments and natural supplements, offering a tapestry of therapeutic therapies for individuals seeking relief from the shackles of chronic pain. In this chapter, we delve into the field of herbal medicine, investigating the rich tapestry of botanical allies and their deep therapeutic advantages.

From time-honored traditions to modern research, we unravel the mysteries of herbal treatments, navigating the roads to safe and effective pain management with clarity, compassion, and appreciation for the wisdom of nature.

An overview of herbal medicine for pain relief

Herbal medicine, steeped in ancient traditions and folk wisdom, offers a comprehensive approach to pain reduction, using the healing power of plants to address the core causes of suffering and imbalance. At its foundation, herbal medicine emphasizes the interconnectedness of body, mind, and spirit, viewing pain not just as a physical symptom but as a sign of deeper imbalances within the body's intrinsic healing mechanisms. By applying a varied array of plant treatments, herbalists strive to restore harmony and energy to the body, helping clients on a journey towards improved well-being and resilience.

Commonly Used Herbs and Their Benefits

Within the field of herbal medicine, a wealth of plant friends stand ready to provide their healing gifts to those in need. From the bright petals of chamomile to the pungent leaves of peppermint, each herb offers its own unique profile of medicinal characteristics, delivering relief from pain, inflammation, and tension. Among the most commonly utilized plants for pain treatment are:

1. Turmeric: renowned for its significant anti-inflammatory effects, turmeric has long been cherished as a natural cure for illnesses such as arthritis, fibromyalgia, and chronic pain.

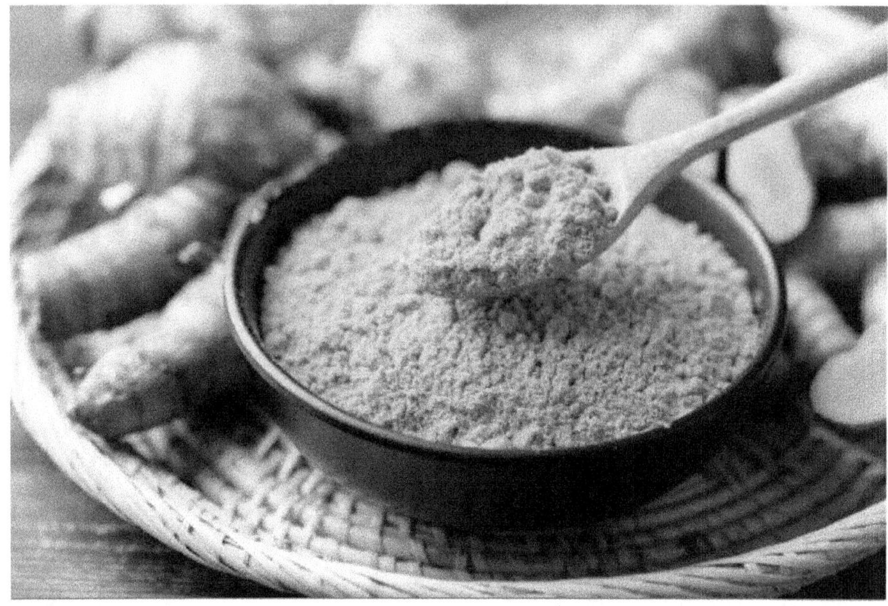

2. Ginger: renowned for its warming characteristics and capacity to reduce stomach problems, ginger also has anti-inflammatory benefits that can help alleviate pain and stiffness.

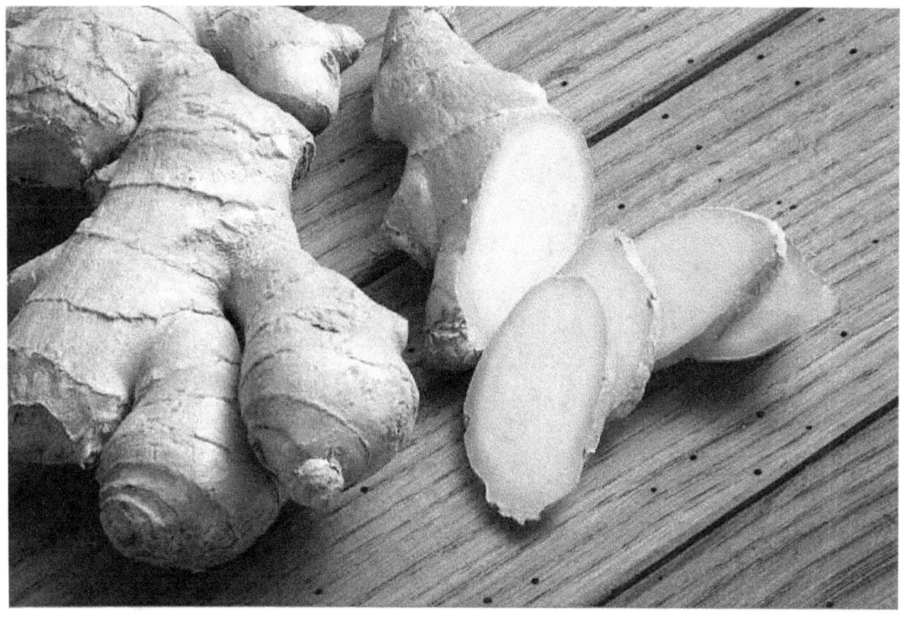

3. Valerian: renowned for its calming characteristics, valerian root is commonly used to alleviate tension, improve relaxation, and enhance sleep quality, making it a helpful ally for people battling with chronic pain-related sleeplessness.

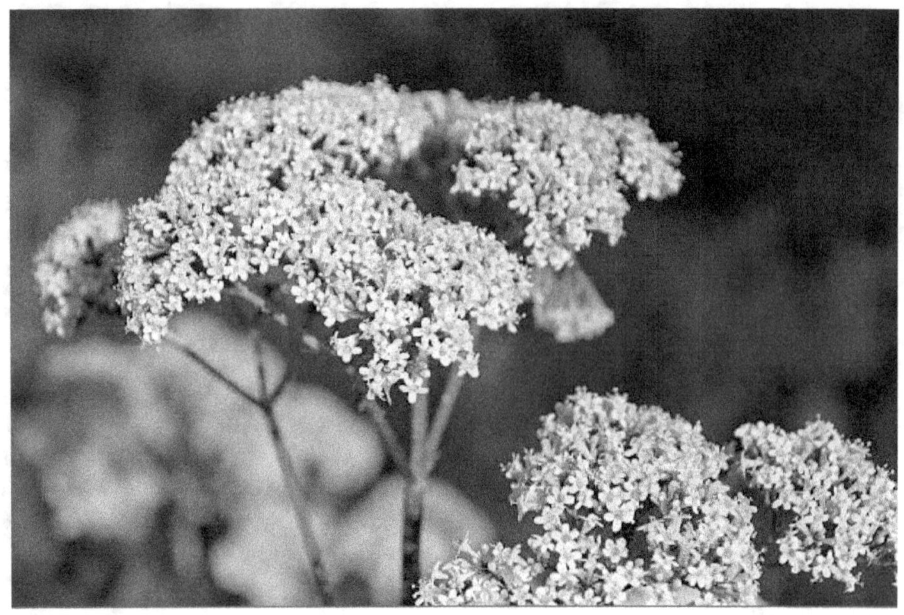

4. White Willow Bark: contains salicin, a chemical comparable to aspirin. White Willow Bark is renowned for its analgesic and anti-inflammatory effects, making it an effective natural alternative to conventional pain medicines.

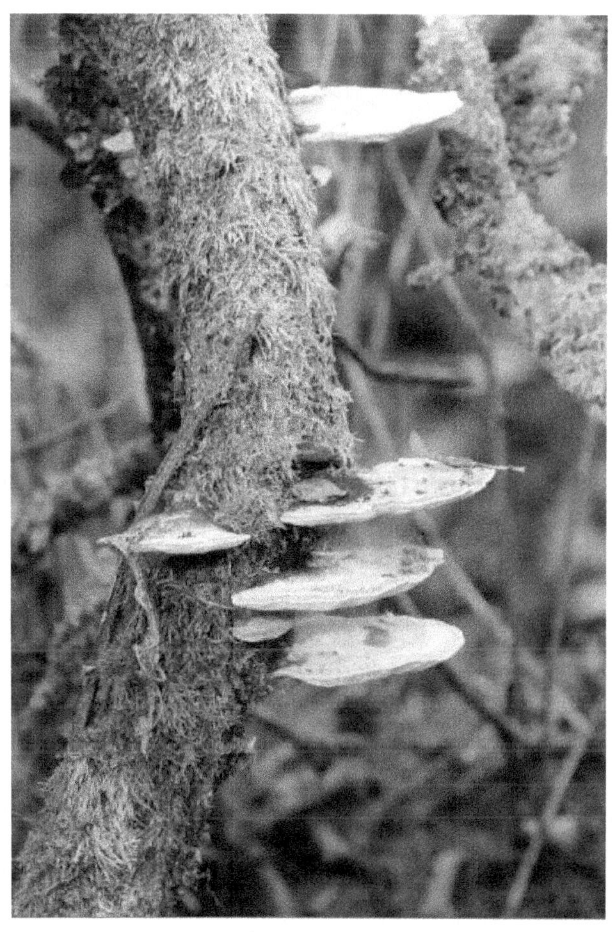

<u>Safety considerations and proper use of herbal remedies</u>

While herbal medicines provide intriguing possibilities for pain alleviation, it is vital to approach their administration with caution and respect for their strong effects. Before commencing on a herbal regimen, persons should speak with a skilled healthcare practitioner or herbalist to ensure safe and proper consumption, particularly if they are pregnant, nursing, or using drugs.

Furthermore, it is critical to select high-quality herbs from reputable vendors and carefully follow dosage recommendations to avoid adverse reactions or interactions. By establishing a mindful and informed attitude toward herbal medicine, individuals can harness the healing power of nature to find relief from chronic pain and embark on a journey towards increased vitality and well-being.

CHAPTER 5

ACUPUNCTURE AND ACUPRESSURE

In the ancient fabric of Traditional Chinese Medicine (TCM), acupuncture and acupressure appear as bright threads, weaving together the profound wisdom of millennia-old healing traditions. Within the soft touch of a needle or the strong push of a finger lies the possibility for profound transformation, bringing peace to individuals traversing the labyrinthine pathways of chronic pain.

In this chapter, we begin on a journey into the heart of TCM, studying the intricate meridians of the body, the art of acupuncture, and the healing touch of acupressure, illuminating routes to relief with clarity, compassion, and reverence for the ancient healing arts.

Understanding Traditional Chinese Medicine (TCM) Principles

At the heart of Traditional Chinese Medicine (TCM) lies a profound knowledge of the interdependence of body, mind, and spirit, viewing health not only as the absence of sickness but as a condition of dynamic balance and harmony. Central to TCM theory is the concept of qi (pronounced "chee"), the essential life energy that flows through the body's meridian pathways, nourishing organs, tissues, and systems. When qi gets stagnant or imbalanced, disharmony occurs, giving birth to symptoms of pain, discomfort, and illness. Through the lens of TCM, pain is considered a manifestation of blocked or disrupted qi flow, suggesting the need for interventions to restore balance and flow within the body's energetic pathways.

Acupuncture: How It Works and What to Expect

Acupuncture, one of the signature methods of TCM, offers a time-honored approach to pain management, using the exact insertion of small needles along specific meridian points to restore balance and flow inside the body. Rooted in ancient Chinese philosophy and informed by modern research, acupuncture is believed to boost the body's inherent healing mechanisms, encouraging the production of endorphins, neurotransmitters, and other biochemical mediators of pain relief.

During an acupuncture session, individuals may experience a sense of deep relaxation, warmth, or tingling when the needles are inserted, followed by a profound sense of relief as stagnated qi begins to flow freely once again.

Acupressure Techniques for Pain Relief at Home

For people seeking treatment for chronic pain in the comfort of their own homes, acupressure offers a gentle yet potent alternative to acupuncture, utilizing forceful pressure on specific acupoints to encourage relaxation, reduce tension, and alleviate suffering.

By applying pressure to specified locations in the body's meridians, individuals can promote the flow of qi, encouraging the body's innate healing processes to alleviate pain and imbalance. From the soothing strokes of a massage to the exact pressure of a fingertip, acupressure techniques can be readily integrated into everyday self-care routines, offering a formidable tool for treating chronic pain with elegance and efficacy.

As we explore deeper into the domain of TCM, we uncover a profound tapestry of therapeutic methods, each offering its own unique pathway to comfort and restoration. Through the delicate touch of acupuncture needles and the compassionate embrace of acupressure, individuals can awaken the body's intrinsic ability for healing, finding peace and sanctuary amidst the ebb and flow of life's currents.

CHAPTER 6

MASSAGE THERAPY AND BODYWORK

In the delicate caress of trained hands lies the promise of release a sanctuary where tension melts away and pain surrenders to the healing touch of massage treatment. In this chapter, we delve into the transforming potential of massage and bodywork, exploring its various advantages for chronic pain treatment, the varied array of methods accessible, and practical tactics for incorporating self-massage into your daily routine.

From the soothing strokes of Swedish massage to the targeted pressure of deep tissue treatment, we go on a journey of healing and rejuvenation, guided by the intuitive wisdom of touch and the endless potential for transformation it holds.

Benefits of Massage for Chronic Pain Management

Massage therapy serves as a beacon of hope for people navigating the labyrinthine pathways of chronic pain, bringing respite from the persistent grasp of tension, discomfort, and dysfunction. Beyond its power to relieve aching muscles and ease tension, massage has been demonstrated to generate deep physiological responses, including the release of endorphins, serotonin, and other neurotransmitters associated with pain alleviation and relaxation.

By increasing circulation, lowering inflammation, and stimulating the release of muscular adhesions, massage therapy provides a holistic approach to pain management, addressing both the physical and emotional elements of discomfort with elegance and efficacy.

<u>Different types of massage techniques</u>

Within the broad tapestry of massage treatment lay a multiplicity of techniques, each giving its own distinct approach to pain reduction and relaxation. From the smooth, flowing strokes of Swedish massage to the targeted pressure of deep tissue therapy, clients can explore a broad variety of techniques adapted to their own needs and preferences. Shiatsu, Thai massage, myofascial release, and trigger point therapy are just a few examples of the rich tapestry of bodywork traditions accessible, each giving its own distinct blend of methods and philosophies to promote healing, balance, and well-being.

<u>Incorporating Self-Massage into Your Pain Management Routine</u>

While professional massage treatment offers a deep avenue for healing, self-massage encourages individuals to take an active role in their own pain management journey, promoting a sense of agency, autonomy, and self-care. By practicing simple self-massage techniques, individuals can address areas of tension and discomfort in the comfort of their own homes, using their hands, fingers, or specialized tools to remove muscular adhesions, increase circulation, and induce relaxation. From foam rolling and tennis ball massage to the mild pressure of self-shiatsu, self-massage offers a varied and accessible approach to pain management, empowering individuals to recover agency over their bodies and their well-being.

As we venture deeper into the realm of massage therapy and bodywork, we encounter a world of unlimited possibility, where healing emerges in the delicate dance of touch and the profound wisdom of the body. Through the caring embrace of experienced hands and the transformational power of self-care, individuals can find refuge, sanctuary, and regeneration amidst the ebb and flow of life's currents.

CHAPTER 7

CHIROPRACTIC ACRE AND SPINAL MANIPULATION

In the complicated web of bones, muscles, and nerves that form the human body lies the delicate balance of alignment and function a symphony of movement choreographed by the spine. In this chapter, we delve into the area of chiropractic care and spinal manipulation, covering the vital role it plays in pain management, the varied array of techniques performed, and essential considerations for locating a trained chiropractor and navigating treatment alternatives.

From the mild adjustments of spinal manipulation to the comprehensive approach of chiropractic care, we begin on a journey of healing and alignment, guided by the profound wisdom of the body and the transformational potential of hands-on therapy.

The Role of Chiropractic Care in Pain Management

Chiropractic therapy stands as a cornerstone of holistic health and wellness, delivering a non-invasive and drug-free approach to pain management centered on the belief that optimal health begins with a properly aligned spine. Central to the practice of chiropractic care is the concept of subluxation a misalignment of the vertebrae believed to inhibit nerve function and damage the body's intrinsic capacity for self-healing.

Through focused adjustments and manipulations, chiropractors strive to restore appropriate alignment to the spine, reduce nerve interference, and promote optimal function throughout the body. From back pain and neck discomfort to headaches, sciatica, and beyond, chiropractic care offers a complete approach to pain reduction, addressing the underlying causes of dysfunction rather than merely concealing symptoms.

Spinal Manipulation Techniques and Their Efficacy

At the heart of chiropractic care lies the art and science of spinal manipulation a hands-on therapy aimed at restoring appropriate alignment to the spine and reducing pain and dysfunction. Through careful and controlled adjustments, chiropractors apply light pressure to specific vertebrae, coaxing them back into alignment and easing strain on surrounding nerves and tissues.

Treatments may vary greatly based on the individual's condition, preferences, and the chiropractor's training and experience, spanning manual adjustments, instrument-assisted manipulation, and gentle traction treatments. While research on the efficacy of spinal manipulation for pain management is ongoing, multiple studies have proved its usefulness in reducing symptoms of low back pain, neck pain, and some types of headaches, providing a safe and effective alternative to more invasive therapies.

Finding a Qualified Chiropractor and Understanding Treatment Options

As with any healthcare provider, locating a certified chiropractor is vital to ensuring safe and effective treatment. When seeking chiropractic care, individuals should prioritize practitioners who are licensed, experienced, and well-trained in the latest techniques and best practices. Personal referrals, online reviews, and consultations can all be excellent resources for discovering competent chiropractors in your region.

Additionally, it's crucial to talk freely with your chiropractor about your symptoms, concerns, and treatment goals, allowing for a collaborative and tailored approach to care. Together, you and your chiropractor can explore a number of treatment methods, including spinal adjustments, soft tissue therapy, rehabilitative exercises, and lifestyle modifications, to construct a comprehensive plan tailored to your particular requirements and preferences.

As we venture deeper into the domain of chiropractic care and spinal manipulation, we encounter a world of potential, where healing emerges in the soft touch of skilled hands and a profound understanding of the body. Through the transformational power of alignment and the compassionate guidance of experienced practitioners,

individuals can discover relief, restoration, and renewed vitality on their journey toward optimal health and well-being.

CHAPTER 8

HEAT AND COLD THERAPY

In the area of pain management, the traditional cures of heat and cold stand as ageless companions, providing natural and accessible methods for reducing discomfort and inflammation.

In this chapter, we investigate the therapeutic benefits of heat and cold therapy, diving into the science behind these time-honored practices, techniques for safe and effective application, and strategies for integrating heat and cold into your specific pain management plan. From the comforting warmth of heat packs to the energizing chill of ice packs, we find the transforming power of temperature modulation and its tremendous impact on the road toward healing and relief.

<u>Using Heat and Cold to Alleviate Pain and Inflammation</u>

Heat and cold treatment represents a cornerstone of natural pain relief, using the fundamental capabilities of temperature to calm tight muscles, reduce inflammation, and promote healing. Heat therapy, which involves applying warmth to affected areas, works by improving blood flow, relaxing muscles, and relieving stiffness and tension a welcome break for people battling chronic pain problems such as arthritis, fibromyalgia, and muscular strains.

Cold therapy, on the other hand, involves the application of cold packs or ice to injured or inflamed areas, constricting blood vessels, numbing nerve endings, and reducing swelling and inflammation an invaluable tool for managing acute injuries, post-operative pain, and inflammatory conditions like tendonitis and bursitis. Whether you're seeking relief from the throes of muscle tension or the flaming tendrils of inflammation, heat and cold treatments offer varied and efficient alternatives for restoring comfort and function to weary bodies.

Techniques for safe and effective heat and cold therapy

While heat and cold therapy offer various benefits for pain relief and inflammation reduction, it's crucial to apply these modalities cautiously and effectively to maximize their efficacy and reduce the danger of damage. When employing heat therapy, select moist heat sources such as warm baths, heating pads, or warm towels, applying them for durations of 15 to 20 minutes at a time to avoid overheating or burns. Similarly, when applying cold therapy, wrap ice packs or cold packs in a thin cloth to protect the skin and restrict exposure to 15 to 20 minutes per session, allowing for enough rest intervals between applications to prevent frostbite or tissue damage. Additionally, it's vital to modify the intensity and duration of heat and cold therapy to fit individual preferences and tolerances, listening intently to your body's signals and adjusting as needed to ensure safe and comfortable treatment.

Integrating Heat and Cold into Your Pain Management Plan

As with any therapeutic modality, the key to harnessing the full potential of heat and cold therapy rests in its integration into a complete pain management plan suited to your particular needs and preferences. Begin by speaking with your healthcare professional to discover the most effective applications and procedures for your unique situation, taking into account aspects such as the nature of your pain, any underlying health concerns, and your overall treatment goals.

From there, explore a range of heat and cold therapy alternatives, including hot baths, warm compresses, cold packs, and contrast baths, to find which techniques resonate most profoundly with your body and bring the best comfort. Finally, consider incorporating heat and cold therapy into your daily self-care routine, weaving moments of warmth and chill into the fabric of your day to nourish and support your body's natural healing processes.

As we embark on this journey through the domain of heat and cold treatment, we discover a world of healing and rebirth, where the transformational power of temperature modulation brings consolation and relief to weary bodies and spirits alike. Through the thoughtful application of heat and cold, we tap into the ancient knowledge of the elements, finding comfort, resilience, and restoration on the path toward optimal health and well-being.

CHAPTER 9

AROMATHERAPY AND ESSENTIALS OILS

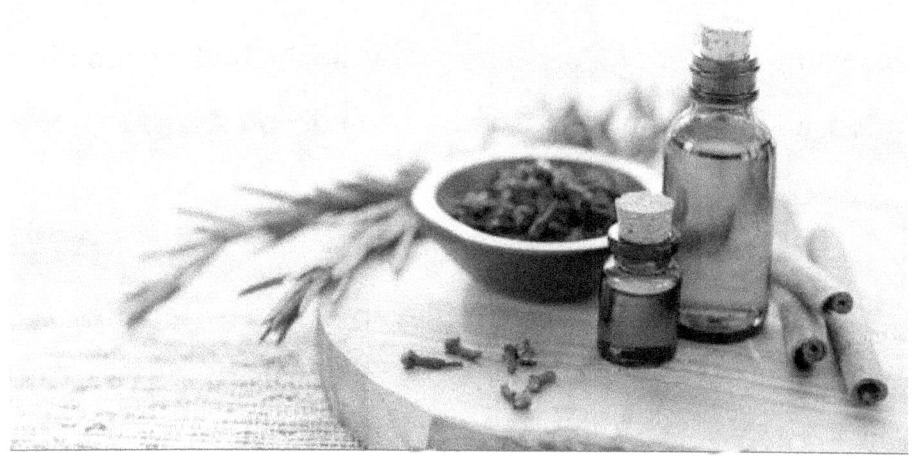

In the realm of holistic healing, the gentle attraction of aromatherapy and essential oils beckons, providing a fragrant gateway to comfort and rejuvenation. In this chapter, we start on a sensory voyage into the realm of

aromatherapy, studying its origins, benefits, and practical applications for pain management and overall well-being.

From the calming embrace of lavender to the stimulating zest of peppermint, we dig into the olfactory riches of nature, revealing their strong capacity to soothe the body, calm the mind, and restore balance to body, mind, and spirit.

Introduction to Aromatherapy and Its Benefits

Aromatherapy, the art and science of employing aromatic plant extracts, known as essential oils, to enhance health and well-being, traces its roots back to ancient civilizations, where floral smells were treasured for their medicinal benefits and spiritual importance.

Today, aromatherapy stands as a time-honored tradition, acknowledged for its varied variety of benefits, including stress reduction, mood enhancement, immunological support, and pain treatment. By harnessing the power of scent, aromatherapy offers a natural and accessible outlet for self-care, enabling individuals to engage their senses and create a deeper connection to the healing forces of the natural world.

Popular essential oils for pain relief

Within the wide tapestry of essential oils lay a select number noted for their amazing potency in reducing pain and discomfort. Lavender, with its delicate flowery perfume, boasts analgesic and anti-inflammatory effects, making it a cherished ally for relieving headaches, muscle tension, and nerve discomfort.

Peppermint, with its cooling mentholaceous fragrance, offers relief from tight muscles, joint discomfort, and tension headaches, while also delivering a refreshing boost to mental clarity and focus. Eucalyptus, recognized for its energizing scent, functions as a potent decongestant and anti-inflammatory agent, great for alleviating respiratory congestion, nasal pain, and muscular tightness. Additionally, chamomile, rosemary, and frankincense are among the ranks of essential oils recognized for their pain-relieving effects, offering numerous avenues for relief and rejuvenation.

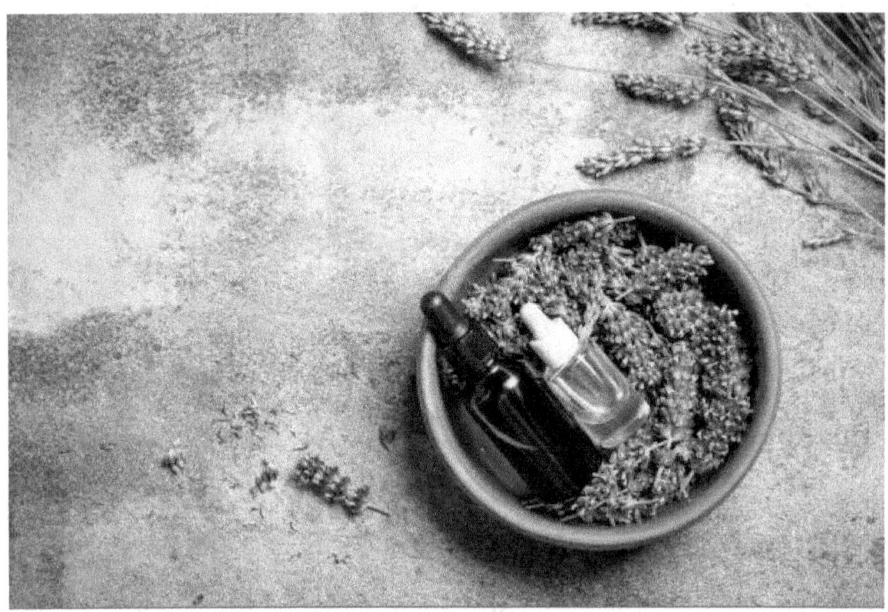

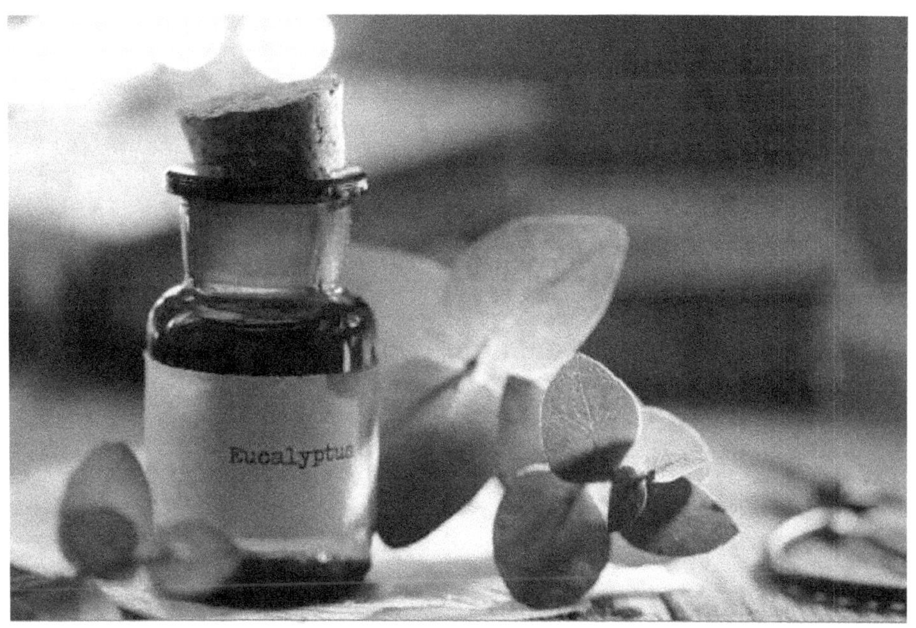

Incorporating aromatherapy into your daily routine

Integrating aromatherapy into your daily routine is an easy and enjoyable undertaking, allowing a plethora of opportunities to permeate your surroundings with the healing aromas of nature. Begin by selecting a few important essential oils that resonate with your senses and meet your specific pain management needs, such as lavender for relaxation, peppermint for invigoration, or eucalyptus for respiratory support.

From there, explore a range of diffusion options, including aromatherapy diffusers, inhalers, or just adding a few drops of essential oil to a warm bath or shower, to create an olfactory refuge in your home or workplace. Additionally, consider mixing essential oils into massage oils, lotions, or handmade balms for topical application, allowing their therapeutic capabilities to permeate deeply into the skin and ease painful muscles and joints. Whether diffused into the air, applied to the skin, or inhaled directly, the transformational power of aromatherapy offers a fragrant gateway to pain relief, relaxation, and renewal, urging you to embrace the therapeutic scents of the natural world on your journey toward wellbeing.

As we immerse ourselves in the captivating world of aromatherapy and essential oils, we discover a realm of sensory joy and therapeutic potential where the aromatic essences of plants serve as effective friends on the journey to healing and wholeness. Through the intentional cultivation of smell, we unlock the healing powers of nature, finding peace, comfort, and regeneration amidst the ever-unfolding tapestry of existence.

CHAPTER 10

MIND-BODY PRACTICES FOR PAIN RELIEF

In the delicate interplay between mind and body lies a tremendous reservoir of healing potential waiting to be accessed. In this chapter, we enter into the domain of mind-body practices, investigating the profound interplay between mental processes and physical sensations and the transforming ability of using the mind to alleviate pain and encourage well-being.

From the mild biofeedback of neural rhythms to the immersive landscapes of guided imagery and the unfathomable depths of hypnotherapy, we embark on a journey of self-discovery and healing, finding the intrinsic potential of the mind to heal the body and restore balance to our lives.

<u>Biofeedback and neurofeedback techniques</u>

Biofeedback and neurofeedback techniques give a window into the delicate workings of the mind and body, allowing individuals to develop understanding and command over physiological processes frequently beyond conscious awareness.

Biofeedback enables individuals to observe and regulate body functions such as heart rate, blood pressure, and muscle tension, allowing them to gain greater awareness and control over their physical responses to pain and stress through the use of sensors and monitoring equipment. Similarly, neurofeedback utilizes real-time feedback of brainwave activity to educate the brain towards states of relaxation and homeostasis, providing a non-invasive and drug-free alternative to pain treatment and emotional well-being. By leveraging the power of biofeedback and neurofeedback, individuals can learn to modify their physiological reactions to pain, improving calm, resilience, and overall vitality.

Guided Imagery and Visualization Exercises

Guided imagery and visualization exercises offer a powerful technique for leveraging the mind's creative ability to elicit healing and transformation inside the body. Through the use of vivid mental imagery and sensory investigation, individuals are led on immersive journeys into imaginary landscapes, where they can tap into their intrinsic potential for relaxation, healing, and self-discovery.

Whether seeing a quiet beach at sunset or visualizing the body's natural healing processes in action, guided imagery allows individuals to access deeper levels of relaxation and inner resourcefulness, generating a sense of calm, empowerment, and resilience in the face of suffering and adversity. By adding guided imagery into their daily routine, individuals can create a profound sense of well-being and completeness, utilizing the power of their imagination to aid healing and restore balance to body, mind, and spirit.

Hypnotherapy for Pain Management

Hypnotherapy, the therapeutic use of hypnosis to aid healing and transformation, offers a gentle yet profound approach to pain management and holistic wellness. By producing a state of profound relaxation and heightened suggestibility, hypnotherapy enables individuals to reach the subconscious mind and examine the roots of their pain, discovering hidden patterns of thought, emotion, and behavior that may be contributing to their misery.

Through the use of hypnotic techniques such as guided relaxation, visualization, and suggestion, individuals can learn to reframe their experience of pain, cultivate greater resilience, and tap into their intrinsic capacity for self-healing and rejuvenation. With the direction of a trained hypnotherapist, individuals can go on a journey of self-discovery and change, unlocking the hidden resources of the mind and awakening to a new paradigm of health, vitality, and well-being.

As we venture deeper into the area of mind-body practices for pain alleviation, we encounter a wide landscape of inner resources and healing potentials waiting to be explored. Through the gentle guiding of biofeedback, the transformational power of guided imagery, and the profound depths of hypnotherapy, we awaken to the intrinsic wisdom of the mind and its capacity to heal the body and restore balance to our lives.

By adopting these practices with an open heart and mind, we embark on a journey of self-discovery and transformation, reclaiming our capacity to heal and live amidst the challenges of chronic pain.

CONCLUSION

As we come to the climax of our journey through the domain of holistic approaches and alternative therapies for managing chronic pain, we stand at the threshold of a new chapter in our healing journey one laden with optimism, perseverance, and the transformational force of self-discovery. Throughout this research, we have delved into the complicated interplay of mind, body, and spirit, revealing a multitude of healing techniques and practices that bring consolation, respite, and fresh vitality to people coping with the problems of persistent pain. In this last chapter, we reflect on the insights gained, the tools obtained, and the route forward towards a life of greater well-being and wholeness.

A Recap of the Holistic Approaches and Alternative Therapies Covered

In our trip through the chapters of this book, we have crossed a broad terrain of holistic methods and alternative therapies, each presenting a unique perspective and set of tools for managing chronic pain healthily. From the mind-body link to the transforming power of nutrition, exercise, and bodywork, we have investigated the varied nature of pain and the numerous ways in which it can be managed holistically. We have dug into the healing possibilities of herbal treatments, acupuncture, and aromatherapy, as well as the tremendous impact of mindfulness, guided imagery, and hypnosis on our perception of pain and well-being. Through each modality and practice, we have witnessed the ability of the human spirit to heal, change, and transcend the constraints of chronic pain, regaining our intrinsic capacity for health, vitality, and wholeness.

Creating Your Personalized Pain Management Plan

Armed with the facts and insights acquired from our inquiry, it is now time to build our individualized pain management plan a roadmap to healing and well-being tailored to our unique requirements, preferences, and circumstances. Drawing upon the principles and techniques described in this book, we can begin to create a comprehensive toolkit encompassing the most effective strategies for managing our pain naturally. Whether it be incorporating anti-inflammatory foods into our diet, practicing mindfulness meditation to cultivate inner calm, or seeking out the support of a skilled acupuncturist or massage therapist, our personalized plan serves as a beacon of hope and empowerment, guiding us towards a life of greater comfort, resilience, and joy.

Moving Forward with Hope and Resilience

As we bid farewell to these pages and continue on the next chapter of our recovery journey, let us carry with us the lessons learned, the insights acquired, and the seeds of hope planted inside our hearts. Let us face each day with courage, resolve, and an unflinching belief in our potential to transcend the confines of pain and live a life of meaning, purpose, and vitality. And let us remember that we are not alone in this journey that we are part of a huge community of other travelers, linked in our shared quest for healing, completeness, and the fullness of life. With hope as our compass and resilience as our guiding light, let us move forward with courage and grace, knowing that the power to heal lies within us, waiting to be liberated and embraced.

As we bring our voyage through the world of managing chronic pain healthily to an end, may we do so with hearts full of appreciation, minds open to potential, and spirits ablaze with the fire of resilience. In the crucible of hardship lies the chance for growth, transformation, and the emergence of a brighter, more vibrant tomorrow. And as we go courageously into that tomorrow, let us do so with hope as our constant companion, guiding us ever ahead towards a life of greater well-being, purpose, and joy